NON-SMALL-CELL LUNG CANCER

EVERYTHING ABOUT NON SMALL-CELL

LUNG CANCER

DR. A. RAMOS

Contents

INTRODUCTION

Approximately 85% of all instances of lung cancer are classified as non-small-cell lung cancer (NSCLC). The reason it is called "non-small-cell" lung cancer is that, when examined under a microscope, the cancer cells are bigger than small-cell lung cancer cells. The most prevalent subtypes of non-small cell lung cancer (NSCLC) include adenocarcinoma, squamous cell carcinoma, and giant cell carcinoma.

Important Information about Non-Small Cell Lung Cancer

1. NSCLC Types:

Adenocarcinoma: This subtype is more common in non-smokers and ex-smokers and frequently starts in the outer regions of the lungs.

Squamous Cell Carcinoma: This type of cancer is usually located in the lungs' central airways and is highly correlated with a history of smoking.

Less frequently occurring, large cell carcinoma can develop anywhere in the lung. It usually spreads and grows swiftly.

2. Reasons and Danger Factors:

NSCLC is primarily caused by smoking, although nonsmokers can also get this kind of lung cancer.

A family history of lung cancer, exposure to secondhand smoke, and environmental contaminants like radon and asbestos are other risk factors.

3. Signs:

NSCLC may not exhibit any signs in its early stages. Common signs of advanced cancer include a chronic cough, chest pain, dyspnea, blood in the cough, exhaustion, and inadvertent weight loss.

4. Conclusion:

A mix of imaging tests (CT scans, X-rays), biopsies, and occasionally molecular testing to detect particular genetic abnormalities or variations are used in the diagnosis process.

5. Setting:

To ascertain the degree of the cancer's dissemination, NSCLC is staged. I stands for localized, and IV for advanced/metastatic. Prognosis and treatment choices are guided in part by staging.

6. Options for Treatment:

The stage and subtype of NSCLC determine the course of treatment. Surgery, radiation therapy, chemotherapy, immunotherapy, targeted therapy, or a mix of these could be available options.

7. Forecast:

The stage at diagnosis, general health, and response to treatment are some of the variables that affect the prognosis for non-small cell lung cancer. In certain circumstances, improvements in therapy and early detection have led to better results.

8. Current Research:

The goals of ongoing research for NSCLC include developing novel therapeutic strategies, immunotherapies, and targeted medicines. There is ongoing research on personalized medicine based on the molecular profile of the tumor.

People who are at danger or who exhibit symptoms must get medical help as soon as possible. The prognosis and available treatment options for non-small-cell lung cancer can be greatly impacted by early detection and prompt intervention.

A broad category of lung tumors that can be further divided into several histological subtypes is known as non-small-cell lung cancer (NSCLC). Large cell carcinoma, squamous cell carcinoma, and adenocarcinoma are the three main subtypes of non-small cell lung cancer. Every subtype is unique and may react to treatment in a different way. An outline of these NSCLC subtypes is provided below:

1. Adenocarcinoma:

Characteristics: The most prevalent NSCLC subtype is adenocarcinoma. It can affect both non-smokers and past smokers, and it frequently starts in the outer regions of the lungs. Adenocarcinoma is more common in women and might manifest as a peripheral nodule or mass.

Histological Features: Adenocarcinoma cells create structures that resemble glands when viewed under a microscope. It is linked to specific genetic alterations, including rearrangements of the ALK gene and EGFR mutations.

Risk Factors: Although non-smokers also frequently develop adenocarcinoma, smoking is still a risk factor. A family history of lung cancer, exposure to secondhand smoke, and environmental contaminants are other risk factors.

2. Cancer of the Squamous Cell:

Features: Squamous cell carcinoma usually starts in the lung's central airways. It is closely linked to a past of smoking.

Histological Features: The flat, thin cells that make up keratin a protein present in skin, hair, and nails are indicative of squamous cell carcinoma. It frequently manifests as a growth or lump in the center.

Risk factors: The main cause of squamous cell carcinoma risk is smoking. Another factor could be exposure to environmental toxins like asbestos.

3. Cancer with large cells:

Features: Compared to squamous cell carcinoma and adenocarcinoma, large cell carcinoma is less prevalent. It tends to grow and spread swiftly and can arise anywhere in the lung.

Histological Features: Since large cell carcinoma does not exhibit the characteristic features of either squamous cell carcinoma or adenocarcinoma, it is diagnosed as an excluding case. The cells have a big, erratic, and undifferentiated appearance.

Risk factors: Smoking poses a serious risk for large cell carcinoma, just as it does for other subtypes of NSCLC.

4. Additional Subtypes:

There are less common NSCLC subtypes in addition to the primary subtypes already discussed, such as sarcomatoid carcinoma and adenosquamous carcinoma. These subgroups have distinct traits and might need different approaches to treatment.

Making decisions about treatment and estimating the behavior of the tumor depend on knowing the histological subtype of non-small cell lung cancer. A more individualized approach to treatment is now possible because to developments in molecular testing, which focus on certain genetic mutations or abnormalities found in the tumor. More subtyping and targeted treatments might become available as research progresses, improving outcomes for those who have non-small cell lung cancer.

A broad category of lung tumors that can be further divided into several histological subtypes is known as non-small-cell lung cancer (NSCLC). Large cell carcinoma, squamous cell carcinoma, and adenocarcinoma are the three main subtypes of non-small cell lung cancer. Every subtype is unique and may react to treatment in a different way. An outline of these NSCLC subtypes is provided below:

1. Adenocarcinoma:

Characteristics: The most prevalent NSCLC subtype is adenocarcinoma. It can affect both non-smokers and past smokers, and it frequently starts in the outer regions of the lungs. Adenocarcinoma is more common in women and might manifest as a peripheral nodule or mass.

Histological Features: Adenocarcinoma cells create structures that resemble glands when viewed under a microscope. It is linked to specific genetic alterations, including rearrangements of the ALK gene and EGFR mutations.

Risk Factors: Although non-smokers also frequently develop adenocarcinoma, smoking is still a risk factor. A family history of lung cancer, exposure to secondhand smoke, and environmental contaminants are other risk factors.

2. Cancer of the Squamous Cell:

Features: Squamous cell carcinoma usually starts in the lung's central airways. It is closely linked to a past of smoking.

Histological Features: The flat, thin cells that make up keratin a protein present in skin, hair, and nails are indicative of squamous cell carcinoma. It frequently manifests as a growth or lump in the center.

Risk factors: The main cause of squamous cell carcinoma risk is smoking. Another factor could be exposure to environmental toxins like asbestos.

3. Cancer with large cells:

Features: Compared to squamous cell carcinoma and adenocarcinoma, large cell carcinoma is less prevalent. It tends to grow and spread swiftly and can arise anywhere in the lung.

Histological Features: Since large cell carcinoma does not exhibit the characteristic features of either squamous cell carcinoma or adenocarcinoma, it is diagnosed as an excluding case. The cells have a big, erratic, and undifferentiated appearance.

Risk factors: Smoking poses a serious risk for large cell carcinoma, just as it does for other subtypes of NSCLC.

4. Additional Subtypes:

There are less common NSCLC subtypes in addition to the primary subtypes already discussed, such as sarcomatoid carcinoma and adenosquamous carcinoma. These subgroups have distinct traits and might need different approaches to treatment.

Making decisions about treatment and estimating the behavior of the tumor depend on knowing the histological subtype of non-small cell lung cancer. A more individualized approach to treatment is now possible because to developments in molecular testing, which focus on certain genetic mutations or abnormalities found in the tumor. More subtyping and targeted treatments might become available as research progresses, improving outcomes for those who have non-small cell lung cancer.

CHAPTER ONE

kinds of lung cancer that are not small-cell

A broad category of lung tumors that can be further divided into several histological subtypes is known as non-small-cell lung cancer (NSCLC). Large cell carcinoma, squamous cell carcinoma, and adenocarcinoma are the three main subtypes of non-small cell lung cancer. Every subtype is unique and may react to treatment in a different way. An outline of these NSCLC subtypes is provided below:

1. Adenocarcinoma:

Characteristics: The most prevalent NSCLC subtype is adenocarcinoma. It can affect both non-smokers and past smokers, and it frequently starts in the outer regions of the lungs. Adenocarcinoma is more common in women and might manifest as a peripheral nodule or mass.

Histological Features: Adenocarcinoma cells create structures that resemble glands when viewed under a microscope. It is linked to specific genetic alterations, including rearrangements of the ALK gene and EGFR mutations.

Risk Factors: Although non-smokers also frequently develop adenocarcinoma, smoking is still a risk factor. A family history of lung cancer, exposure to secondhand smoke, and environmental contaminants are other risk factors.

2. Cancer of the Squamous Cell:

Features: Squamous cell carcinoma usually starts in the lung's central airways. It is closely linked to a past of smoking.

Histological Features: The flat, thin cells that make up keratin a protein present in skin, hair, and nails are indicative of squamous cell carcinoma. It frequently manifests as a growth or lump in the center.

Risk factors: The main cause of squamous cell carcinoma risk is smoking. Another factor could be exposure to environmental toxins like asbestos.

3. Cancer with large cells:

Features: Compared to squamous cell carcinoma and adenocarcinoma, large cell carcinoma is less prevalent. It tends to grow and spread swiftly and can arise anywhere in the lung.

Histological Features: Since large cell carcinoma does not exhibit the characteristic features of either squamous cell carcinoma or adenocarcinoma, it is diagnosed as an excluding case. The cells have a big, erratic, and undifferentiated appearance.

Risk factors: Smoking poses a serious risk for large cell carcinoma, just as it does for other subtypes of NSCLC.

4. Additional Subtypes:

There are less common NSCLC subtypes in addition to the primary subtypes already discussed, such as sarcomatoid carcinoma and adenosquamous carcinoma. These subgroups have distinct traits and might need different approaches to treatment.

Making decisions about treatment and estimating the behavior of the tumor depend on knowing the histological subtype of non-small cell lung cancer. A more individualized approach to treatment is now possible because to developments in molecular testing, which focus on certain genetic mutations or abnormalities found in the tumor. More subtyping and targeted treatments might become available as research progresses, improving outcomes for those who have non-small cell lung cancer.

Reasons and Danger Elements

There are a number of established causes and risk factors for non-small-cell lung cancer (NSCLC), with cigarette smoking being the most significant. It's crucial to remember, though, that people who have never smoked can also develop NSCLC. The main causes of NSCLC and its risk factors are as follows:

1. Smoking:

The primary cause of lung cancer, including nonsmall cell lung cancer (NSCLC), is cigarette smoking. The length of smoking and the quantity of cigarettes smoked each day are directly correlated with risk.

Secondhand Smoke: Breathing in cigarette smoke from other people is a major cause of secondhand smoke exposure, which increases the risk of non-small cell lung cancer.

2. Age:

As people age, their chance of developing NSCLC rises. People over 65 are diagnosed with the majority of cases.

3. Family Background:

An increased risk may result from a family history of lung cancer, indicating a possible genetic predisposition. But shared environmental factors (like smoking habits) within families also matter.

4.   Occupational   and   Environmental Exposures:

Radon Gas: One environmental risk factor for lung cancer, including non-small cell lung cancer (NSCLC), is exposure to radon gas, a naturally occurring radioactive gas that can seep into buildings.

Asbestos: Workplace exposure to asbestos, which is frequently present in industries like shipbuilding and construction, is linked to a higher risk of non-small cell lung cancer.

5. Past Lung Conditions:

People who have a history of lung conditions such as lung fibrosis or chronic obstructive pulmonary disease (COPD) may be more likely to develop non-small cell lung cancer (NSCLC).

6. Personal Background of Other Cancers or Lung Cancer:

Those who have previously experienced lung cancer are more likely to experience another primary lung cancer. The total risk may also be increased by a prior history of other cancers.

7. Genetic Elements:

Although environmental factors are linked to the majority of non-small cell lung cancer cases, research into genetic factors that may predispose certain individuals to lung cancer is still ongoing.

Particular genetic mutations, like those in the EGFR gene, are linked to a higher risk.

8. Gender

Men have historically had a higher incidence of lung cancer. Nonetheless, the incidence of lung cancer in women has increased along with changes in smoking patterns.

9. Ethnicity and Race:

The prevalence of lung cancer varies among various racial and ethnic groups. For instance, compared to White people, Black people typically have higher rates.

It is imperative to acknowledge that although these variables are linked to a heightened likelihood of non-small cell lung cancer

(NSCLC), the onset of the illness is not assured. Furthermore, NSCLC can strike people who have no known risk factors. Managing the risk of non-small cell lung cancer (NSCLC) requires early detection through routine screenings and a focus on minimizing exposure to known risk factors. For individualized advice and monitoring, people should speak with healthcare professionals if they have any concerns or are at a higher risk because of certain factors.

Symptoms and Indications

Non-Small-Cell Lung Cancer (NSCLC) can have a wide range of signs and symptoms, and in its early stages, the illness may not always be evident. As the cancer spreads, people may exhibit the following symptoms and indicators:

1. Chronic Cough:

One common symptom of non-small cell lung cancer (NSCLC) is a persistent cough that gets worse with time. Changes in coughing habits or the onset of a new cough may accompany it.

2. Breathiness Shortness:

Breathing problems or dyspnea may arise when the tumor enlarges and impairs lung function or airways.

3. Pain in the chest:

NSCLC may be indicated by persistent chest pain, which can be dull, aching, or sharp. Back, shoulder, or chest pain are possible locations for the pain.

4. Hemoptysis, or coughing up blood, is:

Coughing up blood or sputum stained with blood can be a worrying sign that lung cancer is present.

5. Weary:

NSCLC may be linked to unexplained weakness or fatigue that doesn't go away with rest, particularly as the cancer gets worse.

6. Unintentional Loss of Weight:

Unintentionally losing a significant amount of weight is a common symptom of many cancers, including NSCLC.

7. Sound of hoarseness

When cancer damages the nerves or structures in the chest, vocal abnormalities like hoarseness may result.

8. Chronic Respiratory Diseases:

Respiratory infections, like pneumonia or bronchitis, that occur frequently or persistently may indicate an underlying lung problem, such as non-small cell lung cancer.

A lung condition, such as non-small cell lung cancer (NSCLC), may be indicated by recurrent or chronic respiratory infections, such as pneumonia or bronchitis.

9. Inability to Swallow (Dysphagia):

If there is an accompanying blockage or if the tumor affects the esophagus, swallowing difficulties may result.

10. Swelling around the neck or face:

If lymph nodes or blood vessels are obstructed by the cancer, swelling in the face or neck may result.

It's crucial to remember that these symptoms are not specific to NSCLC; other illnesses might potentially cause them. Furthermore, in the early stages of the disease, some people with NSCLC might not exhibit any symptoms at all.

It's critical to get medical help right away if any of these symptoms are severe or if there are worries about lung health. Treatment options and overall outcomes can be greatly impacted by early detection and diagnosis of non-small cell lung cancer. Smokers and other high-risk individuals should talk to their healthcare providers about screening alternatives.

Identification and Stage

A number of tests and methods are used in the diagnosis and staging of non-small-cell lung cancer (NSCLC) in order to locate, size, and identify whether the cancer has spread to other parts of the body. The following steps are commonly included in the diagnostic process:

1. Physical examination and medical history:

In order to evaluate overall health and spot possible symptoms, the healthcare professional will obtain a complete medical history, taking into account risk factors like smoking, and conduct a comprehensive physical examination.

2. Imaging Exams:

The lungs are seen and any anomalies are found using a variety of imaging tests:

An overview of the lungs is provided via a chest X-ray.

A CT scan can be used to detect lung nodules, cancers, or involvement of lymph nodes in the chest by providing detailed cross-sectional pictures.

A Positron Emission Tomography (PET) scan can identify possible cancer spread by evaluating metabolic activity in the lungs and other parts of the body.

3. An autopsy

To confirm the existence of cancer and identify its exact type, a biopsy is necessary. A variety of biopsy methods could be employed:

Needle Biopsy: To take a sample of lung tissue for analysis, a thin, hollow needle is utilized.

Bronchoscopy: To obtain lung tissue samples, a thin, flexible tube fitted with a camera is inserted into the airways.

Surgical Biopsy: In certain circumstances, obtaining a bigger tissue sample may need a surgical procedure.

CHAPTER TWO

4. Laboratory Testing:

To find certain genetic mutations or abnormalities inside the cancer cells, molecular testing, including genetic testing, may be performed on the biopsy sample. Particularly for focused medicines, this knowledge aids in guiding treatment decisions.

5. Setting Up:

Treatment choices are aided by staging, which establishes the cancer's degree of dissemination. When staging lung cancer, the TNM method is frequently employed:

Tumor (T): Indicates the main tumor's dimensions and location.

Node (N): Denotes whether lymph nodes in the vicinity have been affected by the cancer.

The term metastasis (M) describes how a malignancy has spread to distant organs.

I (localized) to IV (advanced/metastatic) are the different stages. Additional imaging tests, such as bone scans or brain MRIs, may be necessary for staging in order to determine the degree of metastasis.

6. Tests for Cardiac Function:

Testing for lung function provides information regarding lung function and the effect of a tumor on breathing by measuring lung capacity and airflow.

7. Tests on Blood:

To evaluate general health and spot any anomalies, including liver or kidney function, blood tests may be carried out.

The medical team can then create a thorough treatment plan based on the NSCLC's unique features, such as its subtype, stage, and molecular profile, after the diagnosis and staging are finished. Determining the best course of treatment and enhancing prognoses for those with NSCLC depend heavily on early detection and precise staging.

The management of Non-Small-Cell Lung Cancer (NSCLC) necessitates a multidisciplinary approach, with the selection of a treatment plan contingent upon various criteria including the cancer's stage, subtype, patient general health, and existence of certain genetic abnormalities. The following are typical NSCLC therapy modalities:

1. Surgical:

Resection: This type of surgery removes the tumor together with any surrounding tissue. Various surgical techniques such as wedge resection (removal of a small area of the lung), pneumonectomy (removal of an entire lung), and lobectomy (removal of a lung lobe) may be performed.

2. X-ray therapy:

External Beam Radiation: High-energy radiation is applied from outside the body to the tumor in order to shrink or eliminate cancer cells.

Small, early-stage tumors are frequently treated with highly focused radiation using stereotactic body radiation therapy (SBRT), which is precisely delivered to the tumor.

3. Treatment with chemotherapy:

Chemotherapy medications, which target rapidly dividing cancer cells, are administered systemically throughout the body. In cases of advanced-stage NSCLC, it is frequently administered in conjunction with radiation therapy or surgery.

4. Targeted Intervention:

Medications with Molecular Targets: Targeted treatment seeks to obstruct particular molecular processes that are essential to the development and viability of cancer cells. Treatment options for NSCLC with EGFR mutations include gefitinib, erlotinib, or osimertinib; crizotinib, alectinib, or lorlatinib may be utilized for NSCLC that is ALK-positive.

5. Immunomodulation:

Immune checkpoint inhibitors: Anticancer medications including atezolizumab, nivolumab, and pembrolizumab improve the immune system's capacity to identify and combat cancer cells. They exhibit encouraging outcomes when used in advanced non-small cell lung cancer.

6. Neoadjuvant and Adjuvant Medical Interventions:

Adjuvant therapy is additional care given after surgery to lower the chance of cancer recurrence. It can take the form of radiation, chemotherapy, or targeted therapy.

Neoadjuvant therapy is medication used prior to surgery with the goal of shrinking tumors and increasing the likelihood of a successful surgical excision.

7. Palliative Medicine:

Symptom Management: Palliative care is aimed at easing the symptoms of advanced-stage non-small cell lung cancer patients and enhancing their quality of life. It can be used in conjunction with other therapies.

8. Clinical Exams:

Enrolling in clinical trials could provide access to novel medications and treatments being researched for non-small cell lung cancer.

Based on the unique features of the patient's cancer and the disease, a customized treatment plan is chosen. More specialized and customized treatment modalities are now possible thanks to developments in genetic profiling and molecular testing. People with non-small cell lung cancer

(NSCLC) should be upfront with their medical team about the available treatment options, possible adverse effects, and the overall treatment plan that is customized for them. Results for those with NSCLC can be enhanced by early detection and a thorough approach to treatment.

Way of Life and Assistance Services

Enhancing the overall quality of life and well-being of patients diagnosed with Non-Small-Cell Lung Cancer (NSCLC) is mostly dependent on supportive care and lifestyle choices. Although these actions cannot take the place of medical therapies, they can assist and enhance the therapeutic approach. These are a few facets of NSCLC supportive care and lifestyle:

1. Healthy Eating:

Sustaining general health and preserving strength requires eating a diet rich in nutrients and well-balanced. It is especially crucial to consume enough protein to support the body in meeting the demands of cancer treatment.

2. hydration

Hydration is very important, particularly before, during, and after cancer therapies. Drinking enough water promotes the body's general function and helps handle any possible negative consequences.

3. Moving About:

Regular physical activity can enhance mood, vitality, and general well-being, provided it is done within the individual's capacity. To choose the right fitness regimens, it's crucial to speak with healthcare professionals.

4. Symptom Handling:

Supportive care revolves around the efficient management of symptoms, including pain, exhaustion, and dyspnea. To treat these symptoms, supplementary therapy, medications, and relaxation techniques may be employed.

5. Help on an emotional level:

It can be emotionally taxing to deal with a cancer diagnosis and treatment. To maintain mental health, it is essential to seek out emotional support from friends, family, support groups, or mental health experts.

6. Assistance Units:

People with NSCLC can connect with others going through similar struggles by joining cancer support groups, either in-person or virtually. It may be uplifting and foster a feeling of community to share experiences and coping mechanisms.

7. Assistance for Caregivers:

In the support system, caregivers are also essential. To help them deal with the difficulties of providing care, they might require support and resources. Caregivers might receive emotional support and insightful information from support groups.

8. Sleep hygiene:

It is imperative for persons receiving cancer therapy to establish appropriate sleep hygiene routines. Improved sleep quality can be attained through establishing a cozy sleeping environment and sticking to a regular sleep routine.

9. Supplemental Treatments:

In order to help manage symptoms and enhance general well-being, complementary therapies including massage, acupuncture, and mindfulness training may be helpful. To guarantee these treatments are safe and effective, it's crucial to talk about them with medical professionals.

10. Preparing for Advance Care:

Participating in advance care planning conversations enables people to voice their preferences for care throughout their latter stages of life and guarantees that their desires are honored. Decisions about medical procedures, resuscitation, and palliative care fall under this category.

11. Succession Care:

Maintaining side effect management, tracking treatment progress, and addressing any new issues all depend on routine follow-up visits with medical professionals.

12. Practical and Monetary Assistance:

Seek support for the practical and financial aspects of cancer care, such as resolving logistical issues, negotiating insurance, and gaining access to support programs.

Patients, their support networks, and healthcare providers must work together to offer comprehensive care for people with non-small cell lung cancer (NSCLC). A more patient-centered and holistic approach to controlling NSCLC may be achieved by incorporating lifestyle and supportive care interventions into the overall treatment strategy.

Coping Mechanisms and Emotional Health

It can be emotionally taxing for patients and their loved ones to accept a diagnosis of non-small-cell lung cancer (NSCLC). Here are some coping mechanisms and pointers to encourage mental health:

Embrace Your Loved Ones: Talk to your friends and family about your feelings and concerns. Having a network of support can be consoling and empathetic.

Join Support Groups: Attend support groups for cancer patients to meet people going through similar experiences. It can be helpful to share experiences, and you might learn useful coping mechanisms and insights.

2. Become Informed:

Discover more about NSCLC. Being aware of your diagnosis, available treatments, and possible side effects will help you feel less anxious and be able to make wise decisions.

3. Describe Your Emotions:

Journaling: As an outlet for your feelings and ideas, think about maintaining a journal. Process emotions and keep track of your path through writing, which can be cathartic.

Art & Creative Expression: Express yourself creatively and feel a sense of accomplishment by creating art, music, or writing.

4. Methods of Mindfulness and Relaxation:

Deep Breathing: To help you relax and cope with stress, try deep breathing techniques.

Discover how to be mindful and stay in the present moment by practicing meditation and mindfulness. Resources and apps for guided meditation can be beneficial.

5. Make sensible goals:

Divide Work into Smaller Steps: When faced with difficulties, divide work into more manageable, smaller steps. Honor your progress along the road.

Emphasize Self-Care: Put your health first by eating well, getting enough sleep, and exercising as often as you can.

6. Keep an Upbeat Attitude:

Consider the Present: While making plans for the future is crucial, make an effort to concentrate on the here and now and the things under your control.

Celebrate Little Wins: Give thanks and recognition to little victories and encouraging moments along the way.

7. Talk to Healthcare Providers:

Open Communication: Keep lines of communication open and honest with your medical staff. Discuss any worries, inquiries, and emotional difficulties you may be having.

Request Supportive Services: Make a request for any counseling or psychosocial help that your treatment facility may offer.

CHAPTER THREE

8. Recognize and Welcome Emotions:

Let Yourself Feel: It's acceptable to go through a range of emotions, such as hope, rage, grief, and fear. Recognize these emotions and, if necessary, ask for help.

Professional counseling: To better understand coping mechanisms and emotional stability, think about enlisting the aid of a mental health specialist.

9. Preserve your interests and hobbies:

Participate in Activities: Keep up with the pursuits and pastimes that make you happy and give you a feeling of routine.

10. Attention to Caregivers:

Communication: In addition to seeking help, caregivers should express their emotions. Prioritizing their own well-being is crucial for caregivers.

Respite: To refuel, take breaks when necessary and don't be afraid to ask for help when needed.

NSCLC coping is a journey with both emotional and practical components. Finding coping mechanisms that work for you personally is crucial because every person's experience is different. Connecting with people who have experienced similar things and seeking professional assistance can offer insightful advice and encouragement. Keep in mind that achieving emotional well-being is a continuous process, and it's acceptable to seek assistance when required.

Lifespan and Extended Healthcare

After the first cancer treatment is finished, survivorship in non-small-cell lung cancer (NSCLC) entails addressing the practical, emotional, and physical elements of life. Following NSCLC therapy, the following factors should be taken into account for survivorship and long-term care:

1. Post-Program Care:

To keep an eye on your health, manage any possible side effects, and spot any early warning signs of cancer recurrence, schedule routine follow-up consultations with your healthcare team.

2. Care Plans for Survivors:

Together with your medical team, develop a survivorship care plan that includes information about your past treatments, possible long-term consequences, and a schedule for follow-up care.

3. Taking Care of Late and Long-Term Impacts:

Inform your healthcare staff of any new or recurring symptoms or worries. To preserve wellbeing, it is imperative to address late and long-term impacts such as discomfort, exhaustion, and changes in lung function.

4. Support for Emotional and Mental Health:

Maintain your emphasis on mental health. To address the emotional burden of the cancer experience, seek out counseling, therapy, or support groups if necessary.

5. Healthy Living Options:

A balanced diet, frequent exercise, abstaining from tobacco and excessive alcohol consumption are all important components of a healthy lifestyle. These routines can improve general health and lower the chance of developing further medical conditions.

6. Rehabilitation Programs for Survivors:

Look into physical and occupational therapy-focused survivorship rehabilitation programs. These sessions can help address any lingering issues and enhance and maintain physical function.

7. Counseling on Genetics:

If genetic counseling hasn't already been done, think about doing so to determine your chance of having inherited traits that raise the risk of cancer. You and your family can use this information to guide preventative measures.

8. Financial and Employment Factors to Take Into Account:

During your treatment, take care of any financial difficulties or job changes that may have arisen. To deal with these aspects of survival, look for resources or help.

9. Extended-Duration Monitoring and Screening:

Talk to your healthcare team about screening and long-term monitoring suggestions. Certain tests or screenings may be advised to identify any health issues early on, depending on your treatment plan and personal risk factors.

10. Relationships and Support from Others:

Cultivate ties with loved ones and friends to provide continuous social support. Take part in things that make you happy and give your life a sense of normalcy.

11. Campaigning and Instruction:

Think about stepping up to promote education and awareness about lung cancer. By sharing your expertise and experience, you can help people who are going through similar difficulties by increasing awareness.

12. Preparing for Advance Care:

Evaluate and revise advance care directives as required. Share your choices with family, friends, and healthcare professionals about medical procedures, end-of-life care, and other significant decisions.

Continually adjusting to life after cancer treatment is part of being a survivor in nonsmall cell lung cancer. Keeping lines of communication open with your medical team, attending to issues right away, and taking a holistic approach to wellbeing are all crucial.

Connecting with support networks may foster a feeling of community and understanding, and as a survivor, your experiences and insights can be invaluable resources for others in the cancer community.

Conclusion

To sum up, non-small-cell lung cancer (NSCLC) is a multifaceted illness that necessitates a multimodal approach to diagnosis, treatment, and survival. Along the way, patients and their healthcare teams must overcome a variety of obstacles, from comprehending the risk factors and forms of non-small cell lung cancer to navigating the complexities of staging and treatment methods.

For those with non-small cell lung cancer (NSCLC), improvements in diagnostic methods, immunotherapy, tailored medicine, and targeted therapies provide promise for better prognoses and quality of life. An all-encompassing and personalized approach to disease management is facilitated by early detection through screening and the continuous development of novel medicines.

Beyond medical treatments, it is critical to address the psychological, social, and practical elements of non-small cell lung cancer. Support systems, coping mechanisms, and mental health all play significant roles in assisting people in overcoming the difficulties associated with receiving a cancer diagnosis.

In order to survive NSCLC, a person must accept a holistic approach to wellbeing, manage any potential long-term repercussions, and engage in continuous monitoring. Advances in our understanding of NSCLC and the quality of life for those impacted by this difficult condition are made possible by ongoing research, community support, and advocacy initiatives.

By working together, patients, medical professionals, researchers, and support systems aspire to treat non-small cell lung cancer (NSCLC) more successfully while also improving the quality of life for survivors and giving them hope for the future.

THE END

www.ingramcontent.com/pod-product-compliance
Lightning Source LLC
Chambersburg PA
CBHW060805260726
48660CB00002B/781